HEART DISEASE DIET COOKBOOK FOR KIDS

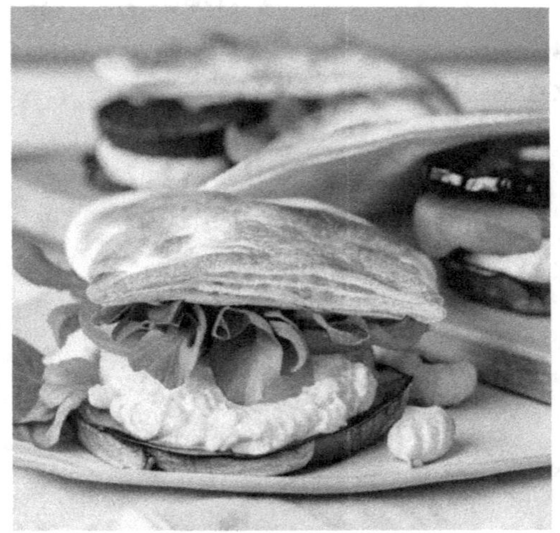

The Ultimate Quick and Easy Delicious Recipes for Children

Jessica Murray

Dear Reader,

Thank you for the purchase. I hope you enjoy and love it, would you consider dropping an honest feedback/review, I will appreciate that and you can contact me using JessicaMurrayDietHelp@gmail.com if you have any questions, I will gladly respond

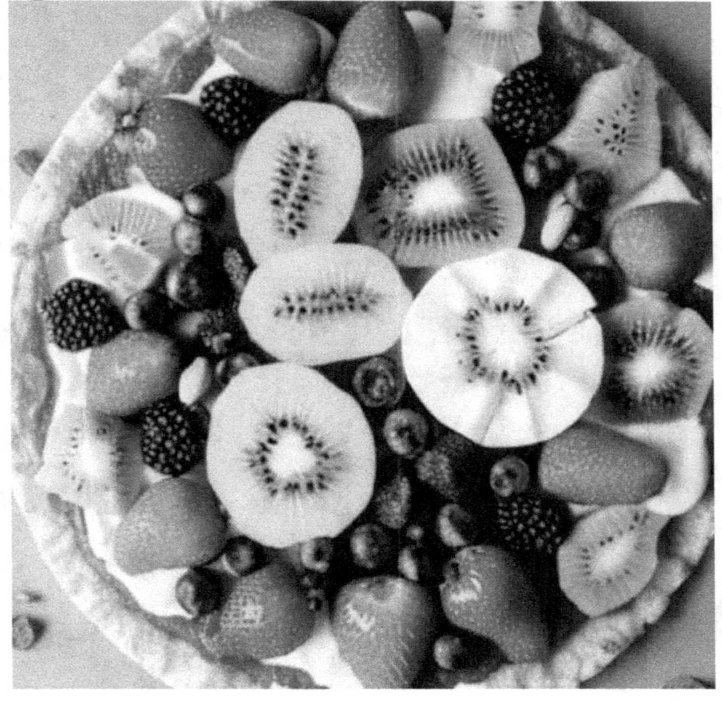

Table of Contents

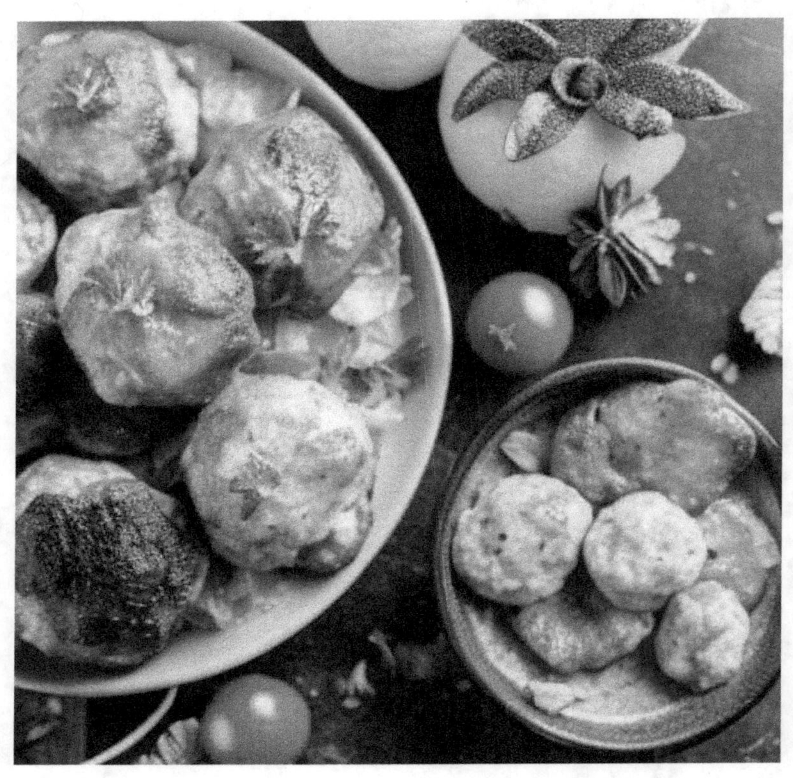

INTRODUCTION

Jason embodied the term "picky eater." He was always so hesitant to try new things and would rather eat the same few meals every single day. Jim and Sue, his parents, were frantic to change his diet for the better, but it seemed that no matter how hard they tried, nothing was ever successful.

Finally, they made the decision to attempt the Heart Disease Recipes Cookbook for Kids in an effort to persuade their kid to eat healthier. Jason was shocked to discover that he enjoyed a number of the recipes in the book despite his initial mistrust. Jim and Sue felt they made the right choice after observing the wonderful effects the cookbook had on the meals their family enjoyed.

Upon tasting the cookbook's delectable recipes, Jason's initial hesitancy quickly disappeared. He started eating more fruits and vegetables and even started developing his own recipes as a result of his newfound enthusiasm for heart-healthy, nutritious food. After a few months, Jason has fully changed from being a finicky eater. He now eats a wide range of heart-healthy, healthful dishes that his parents could only have imagined when they first purchased the cookbook. The family's purchase of The Heart Disease Recipes Cookbook for Kids turned out to be a wise decision, as it was the key to encouraging Jason to adopt healthy eating practices. This cookbook came in handy and transformed the way the entire family views eating thanks to its straightforward, simple-to-follow instructions and delectable recipes.

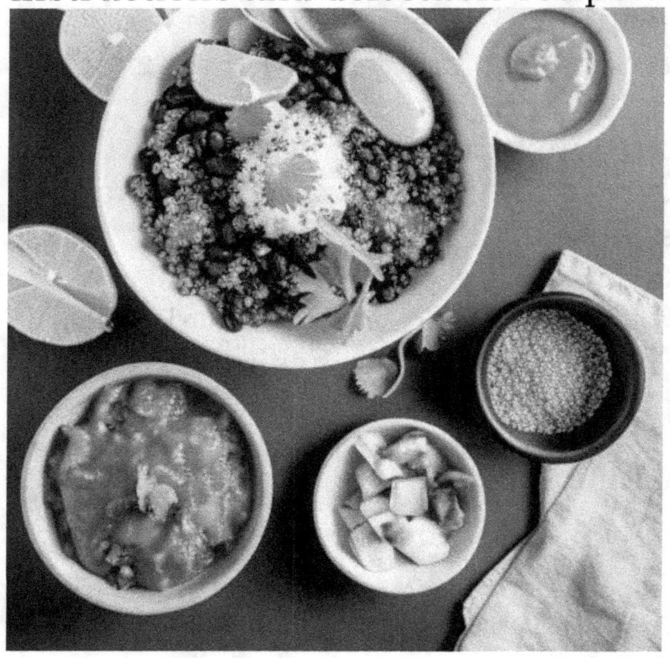

Chili Lime Salmon Burgers

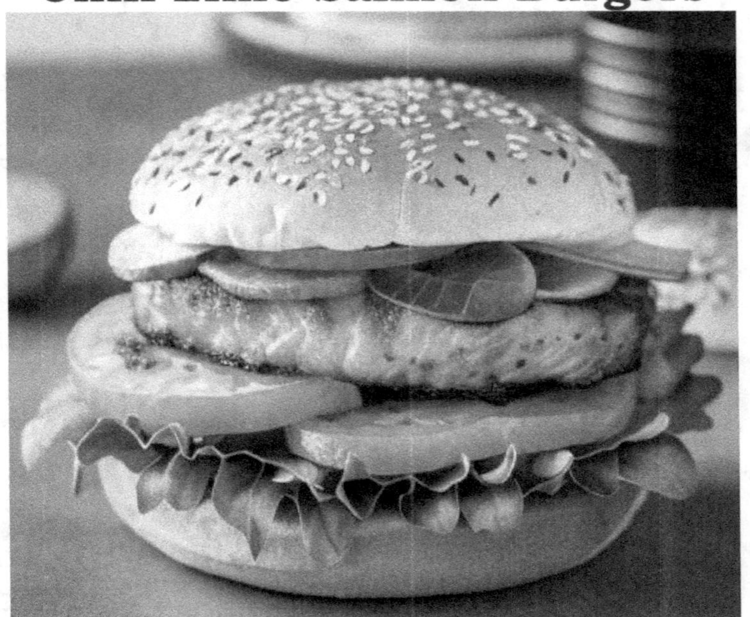

Ingredients:

- 1 pound of wild salmon
- 1/2 cups red onion, coarsely chopped 2 cloves of minced garlic
- 2 teaspoons chopped fresh cilantro
- 2 tbsp. lime juice
- One tablespoon of chili powder1 teaspoon cumin, ground
- To taste, add salt and pepper
- 2 teaspoons Avocado Oil

Instructions:

- Put the salmon in a bowl and carefully separate it into little pieces using a fork.
- Include and thoroughly blend the red onion, garlic, cilantro, lime juice, chili powder, cumin, salt, and pepper.
- In a big skillet over medium-high heat, warm the olive oil.
- Shape the salmon mixture into four to five patties.
- Once the patties are in the skillet, fry them for about four minutes on each side, or until they are fully cooked.
- Top the burgers with your preferred toppings and serve them on toasted buns. Enjoy!

Grilled Shrimp Skewers

Ingredients:

- 2 tablespoons of olive oil and 1 teaspoon of garlic powder 1 pound of peeled and deveined shrimp
- One tablespoon of chili powder
- One lime's juice
- To taste, add salt and pepper.

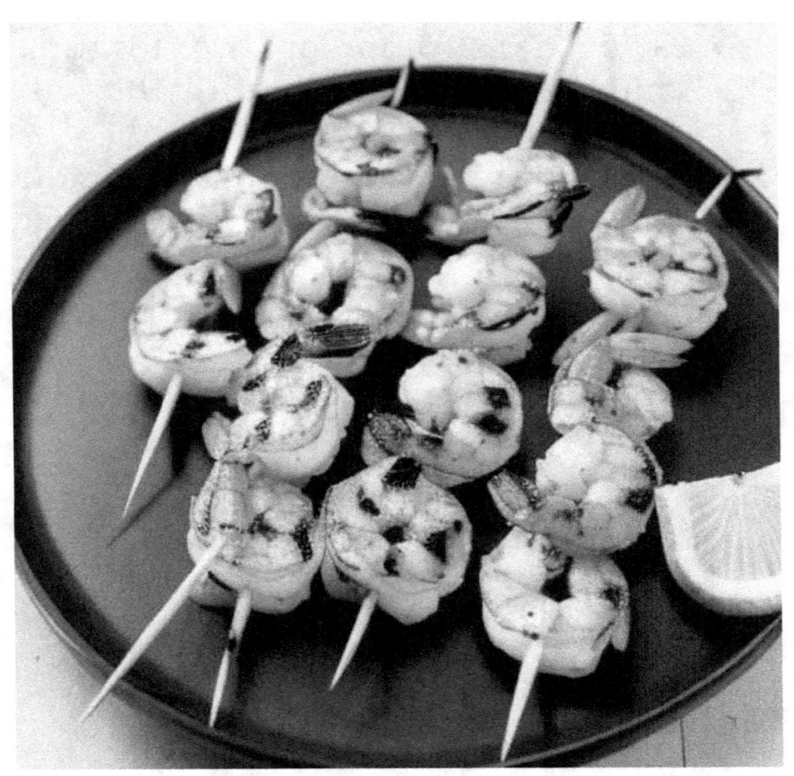

Instructions:

- Turn on medium heat on a grill or grill pan.
- Combine the olive oil, lime juice, garlic powder, chili powder, salt, and pepper in a small bowl.
- Toss the shrimp with the marinade to coat it
- Using metal skewers, thread the shrimp.

- Grill the shrimp for two to three minutes per side, or until they are fully cooked.
- Top with your preferred sauce and a wedge of lime, and serve over a bed of greens. Enjoy!

Avocado and Feta Cheese Toast

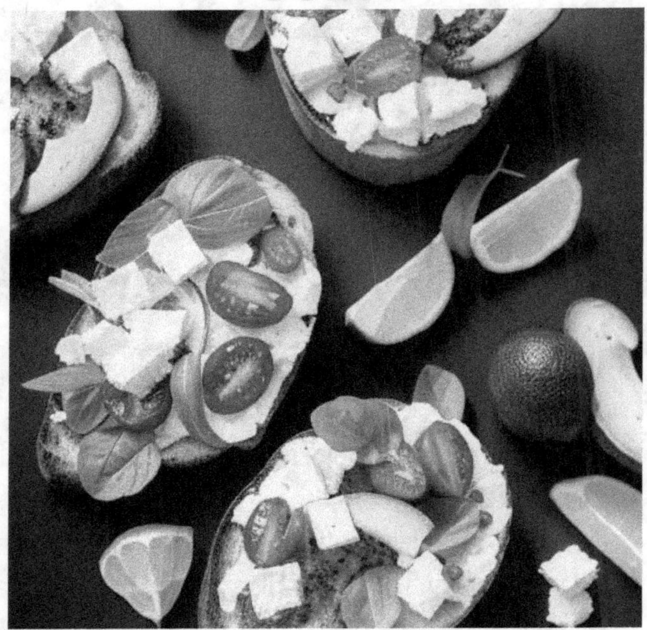

Ingredients:
- 2 slices of multigrain bread; 1 mashed, ripe avocado.
- 1/2 lime juice

- 2 teaspoons of fresh parsley that has been chopped
- To taste, add salt and pepper.

Instructions:
- Toast the bread pieces.
- Combine the avocado, feta cheese, parsley, lime juice, salt, and pepper in a small bowl.
- Apply the mixture to the slices of toasted bread.
- Dish out and savor!

Eggplant & Hummus Pita Sandwich

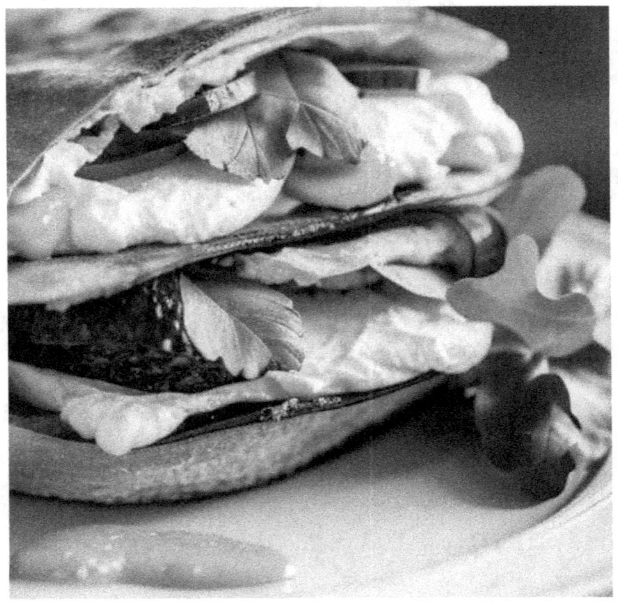

Ingredients:

- 1 large eggplant, cut into rounds about 1/4-inch thick
- Olive oil, 2 tablespoons
- 4 pita pockets; salt and pepper to taste
- A cup of hummus
- One-fourth cup feta cheese
- 1/2 cup freshly chopped tomatoes
- 1/2 cup freshly sliced cucumber
- 1/4 cup freshly chopped parsley

Instructions:

- Turn the heat to medium-high on a grill or grill pan.
- Sprinkle salt and pepper over the eggplant slices after brushing them with olive oil.
- Grill the eggplant slices for a total of 2–3 minutes, or until they are just beginning to brown.
- Split the pita pockets apart, then hummus each one.
- Add the feta cheese, tomatoes, cucumber, parsley, and eggplant slices on top.
- Dish out and savor!

Turkey Sloppy Joes

Ingredients:

- 1 pound of ground turkey,
- 1/2 small yellow onion, 1/2 red bell pepper, and 2 minced garlic cloves
- One-fourth cup tomato sauce
- Ketchup, two tablespoons
- 2 tablespoons of Worcestershire sauce 1 teaspoon brown sugar
- One tablespoon of chili powder
- To taste-adapt salt and pepper, 4 hamburger buns

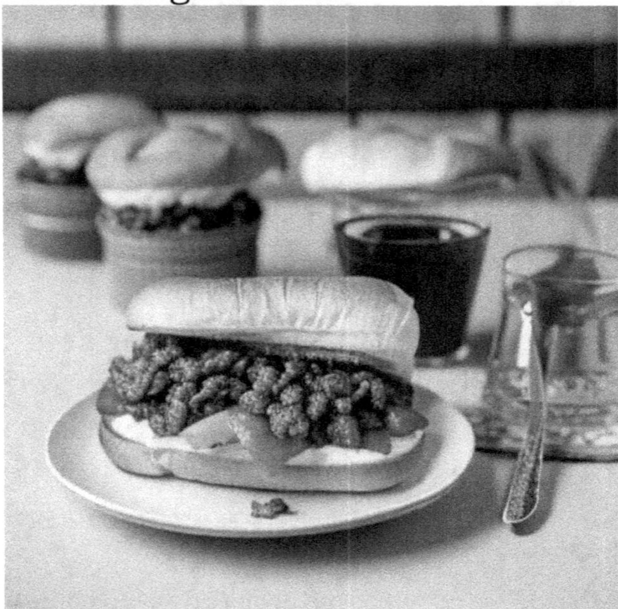

Instructions:

- In a sizable skillet, sauté the ground turkey until thoroughly heated through.
- Include the bell pepper, onion, and garlic and simmer for 2 to 3 minutes, or until the vegetables are tender.
- Include the salt, pepper, brown sugar, chili powder, tomato sauce, ketchup, and Worcestershire sauce and mix well.
- Once the sauce has thickened, continue cooking for an additional 5-7 minutes over medium heat.
- Place the hamburger buns on top of the turkey mixture, and eat!

Quinoa and Black Bean Burrito Bowls

Ingredients:

- 1 cup of quinoa,
- 1 15-ounce can of rinsed and drained black beans, 1 diced red bell pepper, and 1/2 cup of corn kernels
- 1/2 cup red onion, finely chopped
- 2 teaspoons cumin, 2 tablespoons olive oil
- One lime's juice1/2 cup freshly chopped cilantro

- To taste, add salt and pepper.

Instructions:

- Prepare the quinoa as directed on the package.
- Place the bell pepper, corn, red onion, and black beans in a big bowl.
- Combine the olive oil, cumin, lime juice, cilantro, salt, and pepper in a small bowl.
- After adding the dressing to the vegetables, blend them.
- Include the prepared quinoa in the bowl and stir to incorporate.
- Add additional cilantro and your preferred toppings, then enjoy!

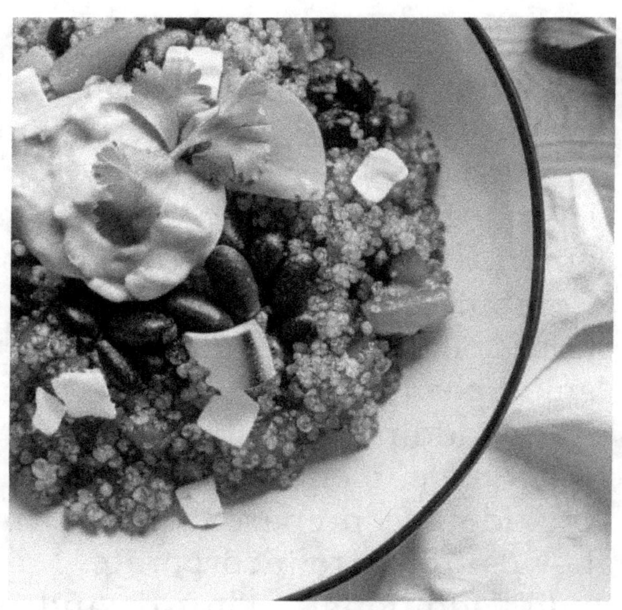

Mediterranean Pizza

Ingredients:
- One ready-made pizza crust and Half a cup of marinara sauce
- 1/2 cup sliced black olives
- 1/2 cup chopped artichoke hearts
- One-fourth cup feta cheese
- 1/4 cup chopped sun-dried tomatoes
- 1/4 cup freshly chopped basil

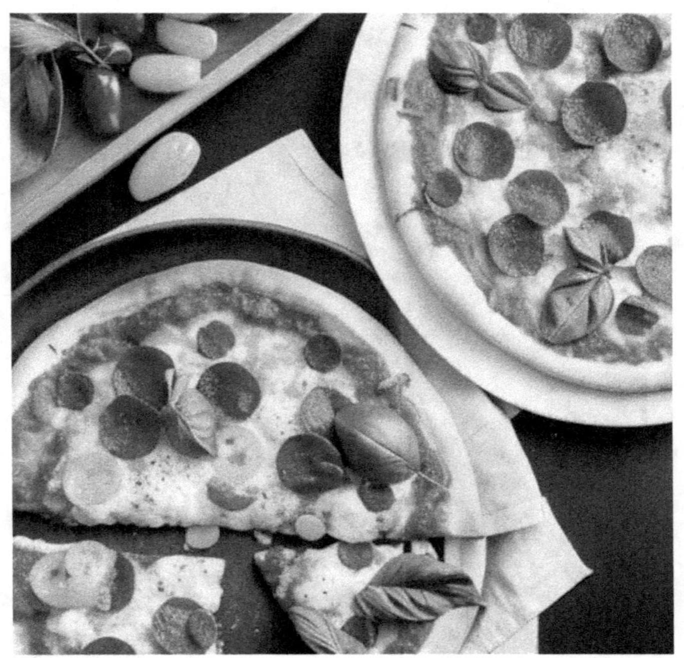

Instructions:

- Set the oven to 450 degrees
- Put the pizza crust on a baking sheet in step two.
- Top the pizza crust with the feta cheese, sun-dried tomatoes, basil, black olives, and artichoke hearts after evenly spreading the marinara sauce over it.
- Bake for 15 minutes, or until the cheese is melted and the crust is golden brown.
- Present and savor!

Lentil Vegetable Soup

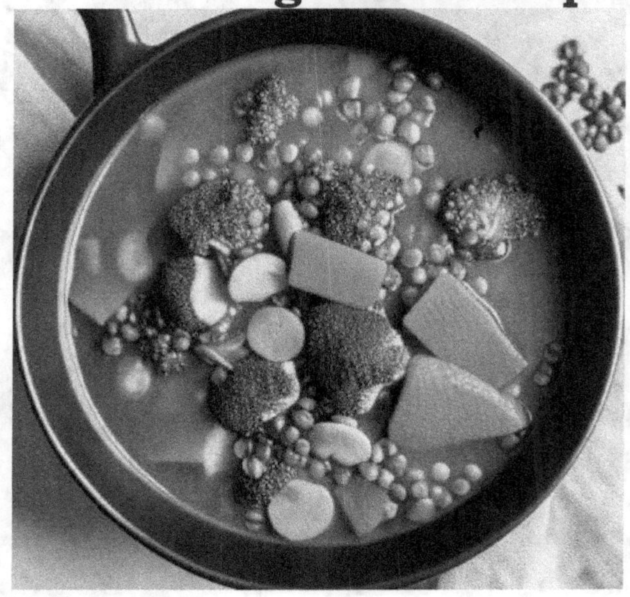

Ingredients:

- 1 tablespoon of olive oil
- 2 minced garlic cloves 1 tiny yellow onion
- 2 sliced carrots
- 2 chopped celery stalks
- 1/2 cup green lentils, 1 can diced tomatoes
- 2 cups vegetable broth
- 1 teaspoon each of dried basil, dried thyme, and dried oregano
- To taste, add salt and pepper.

Instructions:

- In a big pot over medium heat, warm the olive oil.
- Include the celery, carrots, onion, and garlic and simmer for a further 5 minutes, or until the veggies are tender.
- Bring to a boil the lentils, vegetable broth, diced tomatoes, oregano, thyme, basil, salt, and pepper.
- After the lentils begin to boil, lower the heat to a simmer for 20 minutes, or until they are thoroughly cooked.
- Include your preferred toppings in the soup and serve it with a side of crusty bread. Enjoy!

Greek Yogurt Parfaits

Ingredients:

- Greek yogurt, 1 cup
- Honey, 1 tablespoon
- A quarter cup of granola
- Fresh berries Totaling 1/4 cup

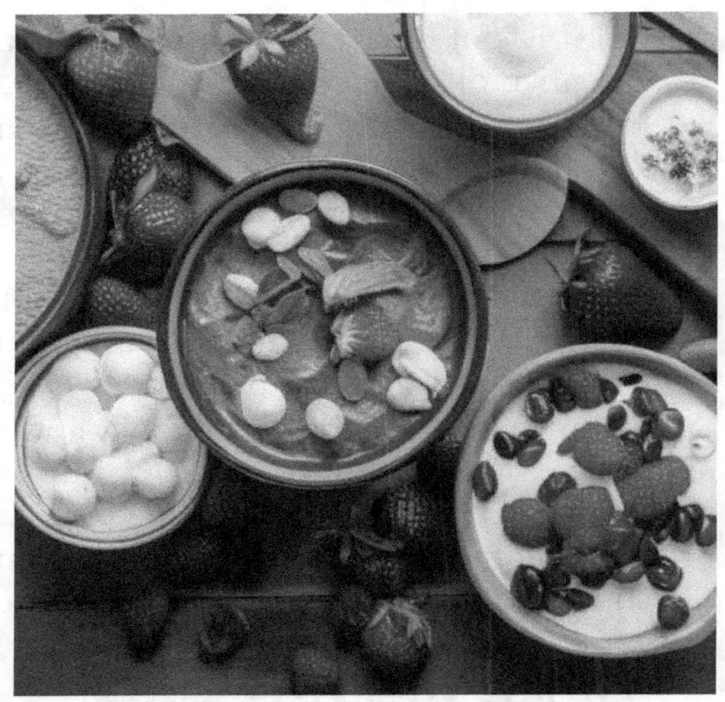

Instructions:

- Begin by placing the Greek yogurt on a bowl's base.
- Drizzle the yogurt with the honey.
- Top the honey with the granola.
- Add berries to the parfait's top.
- Enjoy!

Spaghetti Squash with Tomato and Spinach

Ingredients:

- Spaghetti squash, one

- One teaspoon of olive oil
- onion, diced, 1/4 cup
- 1/2 cup tomatoes, diced
- 2 minced garlic cloves
- 2 cups baby kale
- To taste, add salt and pepper.

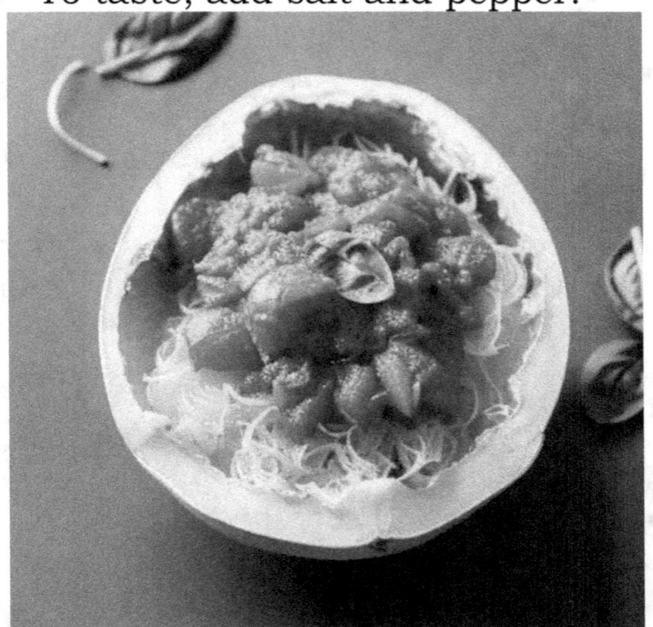

Instructions:

- Set the oven to 425 Fahrenheit.
- Place spaghetti squash on a baking pan after cutting it in half lengthwise.
- After brushing the squash with oil, roast it for 40 minutes.

- After the squash has finished cooking, take it out of the oven and allow it to cool.
- Set a large skillet over medium heat and warm the olive oil.
- Continue to sauté the onion for 3 minutes.
- Include the spinach, tomatoes, and garlic.
- Cook until the spinach wilts and the tomatoes soften.
- Scoop the spaghetti squash strands out of their skins with a large spoon, add them to the skillet, and stir.
- Add salt and pepper, then serve.

Veggie Quesadillas

Ingredients:
- 2 substantial tortillas
- Black beans, 1/4 cup
- 1/4 cups of corn
- 1/4 cup red bell peppers, chopped
- onion, diced, 1/4 cup
- 1 cup of cheese, shredded

Instructions:
- Set a sizable skillet over medium heat to preheat.

- Place one tortilla on the griddle and top with half of the bell pepper, onion, black beans, and corn.
- Add 1/2 cup of the cheese shavings on top.
- Lay the second tortilla on top, pressing down just a little.
- Cook 3 minutes or until the bottom is light brown and cheese begins to melt.
- Turn the food over and cook it for three more minutes.
- Serve after cutting into four wedges.

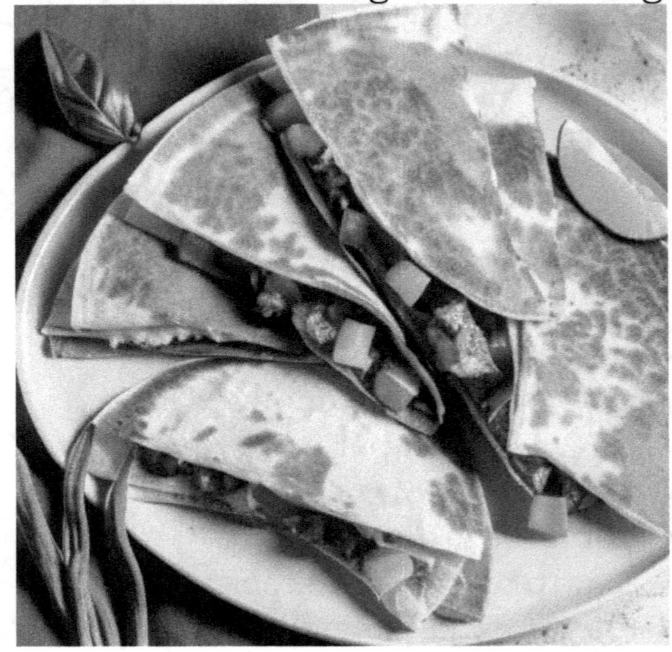

Brown Rice Jambalaya

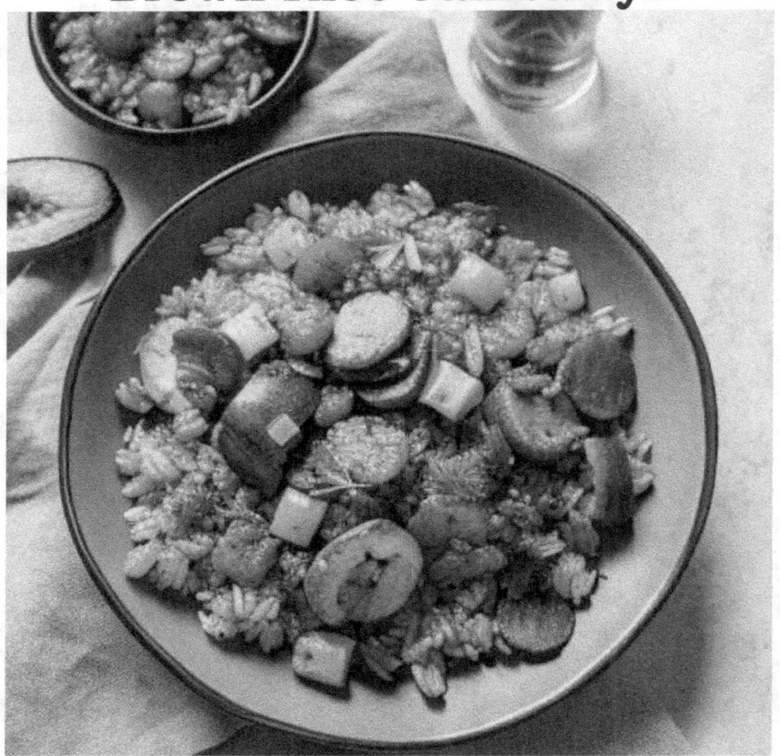

Ingredients:

- One teaspoon of olive oil
- 1 cup of onion, diced
- 1/2 cup celery, chopped
- 1/2 cup bell peppers, chopped
- One teaspoon of garlic mince
- tomatoes, diced, 1 cup
- 1 cup of chicken stock
- Cayenne pepper, half a teaspoon

- smoked paprika, 1 teaspoon
- 1 serving of brown rice
- 1 tsp. oregano
- 2 teaspoons of parsley, chopped
- 1/2 cup finely minced green onion

Instructions:

- In a big skillet over medium-high heat, warm the olive oil.
- Include the chopped celery, onion, bell pepper, and garlic.
- Cook for about 5 minutes, or until the vegetables start to soften.
- Include the tomatoes and boil after adding the chicken broth.
- Add the brown rice, cayenne pepper, and smoked paprika.
- Cook the rice on low heat for about 25 minutes, stirring regularly, until it is fluffy and soft.
- Add the green onion and parsley.
- Dish out and savor!

Baked Salmon with Steamed Veggies

Ingredients:

- 2 salmon fillets, weighing 4 ounces
- To taste, add salt and pepper.
- One teaspoon of olive oil

- 1 cup of carrots, diced
- 1 cup of shredded zucchini
- 1/2 teaspoon garlic, minced

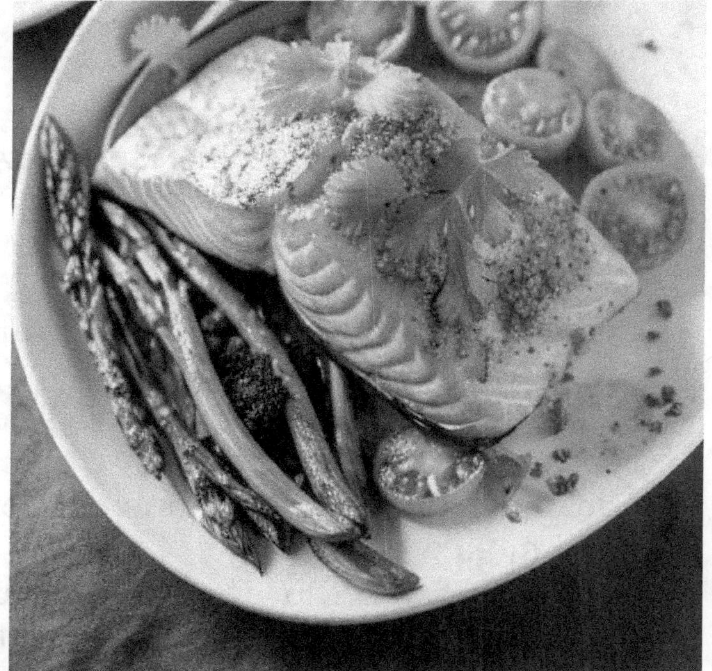

Instructions:

- Set the oven's temperature to 375 F.
- Using a paper towel, pat the salmon fillets dry before seasoning them with salt and pepper.
- Cook the salmon for 3 minutes on each side in a large skillet with the olive oil heated to medium heat.

- Bake the skillet for 10 minutes in the oven.
- In the meantime, steam the zucchini and carrots for five minutes.
- Turn off the oven and add the steamed vegetables to the skillet.
- Include the garlic and whisk to incorporate.
- Present the warm fish and vegetables.

Fruit and Cheese Kebabs

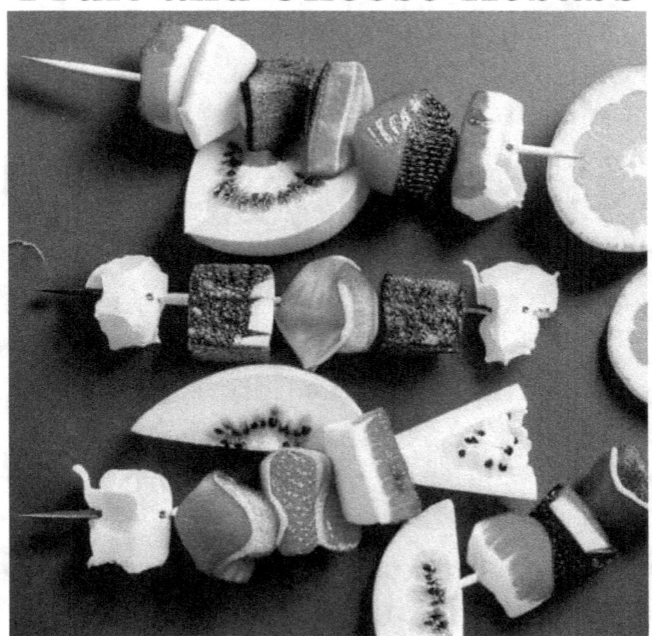

Ingredients:

- 1 cup cubed sharp cheddar cheese and 1 cup cubed mozzarella cheese
- 1 cup of cubed smoked cheese
- 2 cored and cubed apples
- 2 cored and cubed pears
- Eight wood skewers

Instructions:

- Set the oven to 375 degrees.
- Alternate the cheese cubes and fruit cubes on each skewer.
- Arrange the prepared kebabs on a baking sheet that has been oiled.
- To melt the cheese, bake for 8 to 10 minutes.
- Present hot.

Baked Turkey Meatballs

Ingredients

- One egg and one teaspoon of garlic powder.
- One tablespoon of onion powder
- Italian seasoning, 1 teaspoon
- One tablespoon Worcestershire sauce
- 1/2 teaspoon sea salt, 1/2 teaspoon black pepper

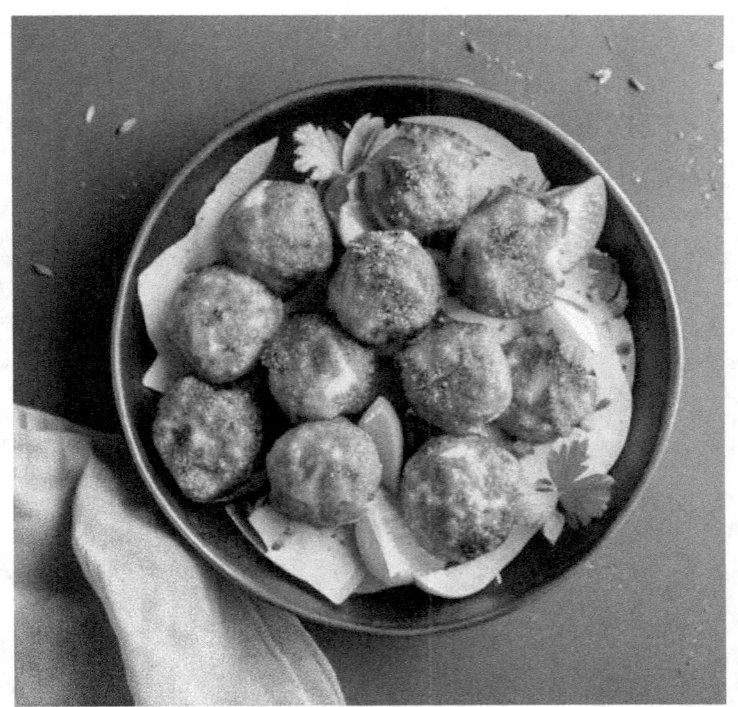

Instructions:

- Turn on the oven to 400°F.
- Combine the ground turkey, breadcrumbs, egg, Italian seasoning, Worcestershire sauce, garlic powder, onion powder, and sea salt in a big bowl. Combining thoroughly after mixing.
- Shape the mixture into meatballs that are 1 inch in diameter.

- Set the meatballs on a baking sheet that has been buttered.
- Bake for 18 to 20 minutes, or until thoroughly heated through.
- Present hot.

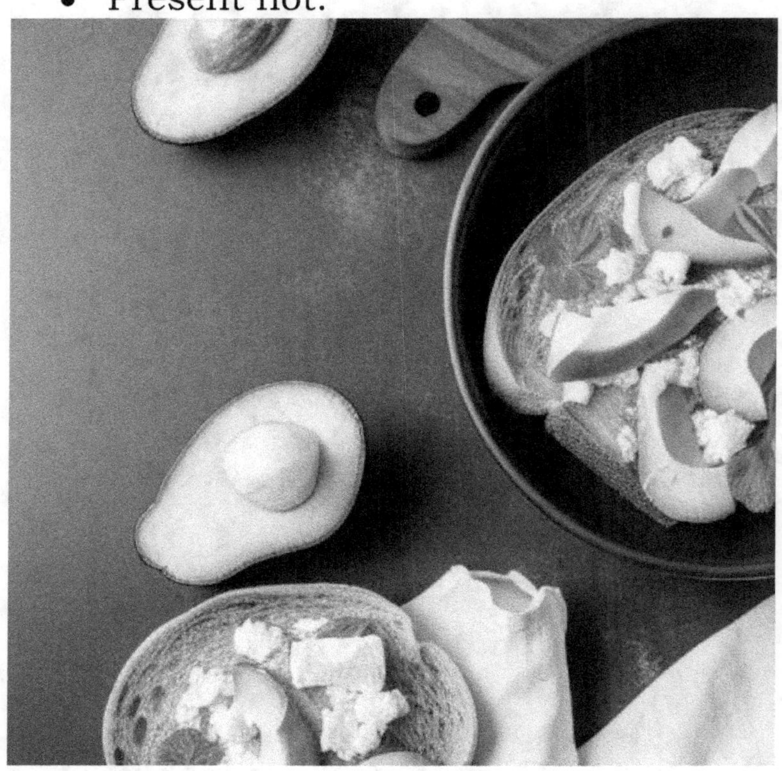

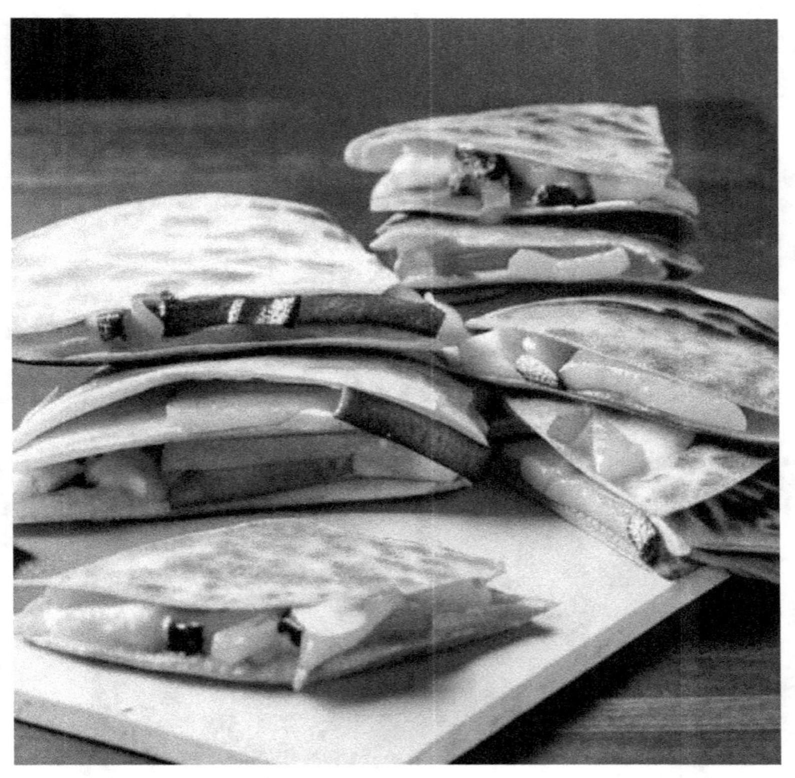

Baked Apples with Raisins and Cinnamon

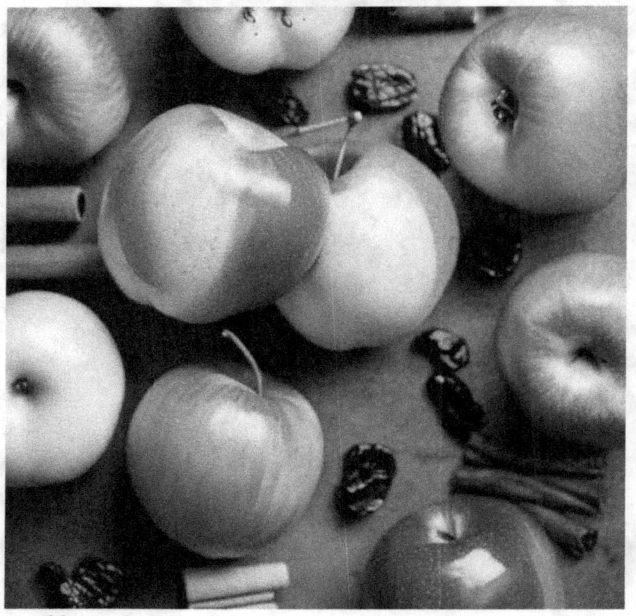

Ingredients:

- four apples
- 1 tablespoon of ground cinnamon
- 2 tablespoons of melted butter
- and 2 teaspoons of dark brown sugar
- A quarter cup of golden raisins

Instructions:

- Set the oven's temperature to 350°F.

- Place the apple slices in an 8-inch square baking dish after coring and slicing them.
- Sprinkle the brown sugar, cinnamon, and raisins on top of the apples, and drizzle the melted butter over them.
- Bake the apples for 25 to 30 minutes, or until they are fully cooked and golden.

Healthy Berry Cobbler

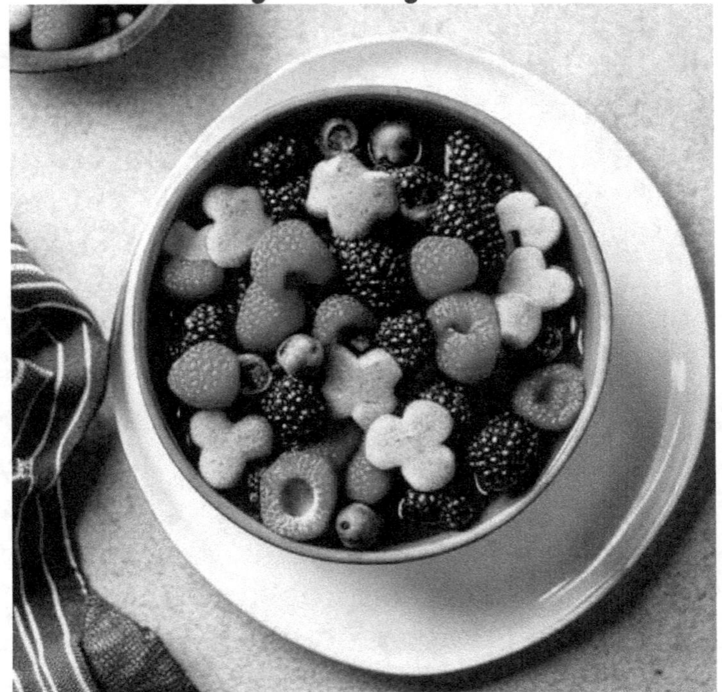

Ingredients:

- 2 cups of berries, either fresh or frozen
- 1 cup of whole wheat flour
- 3/4 cup of oats; 3/4 cup of brown sugar
- and 1/4 teaspoon of baking powder.
- 6 tablespoons of melted butter and 1/4 teaspoon of salt
- 1/4 cup of Greek yogurt, plain

Instructions:

- Set the oven to 350 degrees.
- Use cooking spray to grease an 8-inch square baking dish.
- Arrange the berries evenly in the bowl.
- Combine the flour, oats, brown sugar, baking soda, and salt in another bowl.
- Combine the Greek yogurt and melted butter after adding them.
- Disperse the mixture over the berries' tops.
- Bake for 40 minutes, or until the berries are popping and the top is brown. Before serving, allow it to cool.

Sweet Potato Muffins

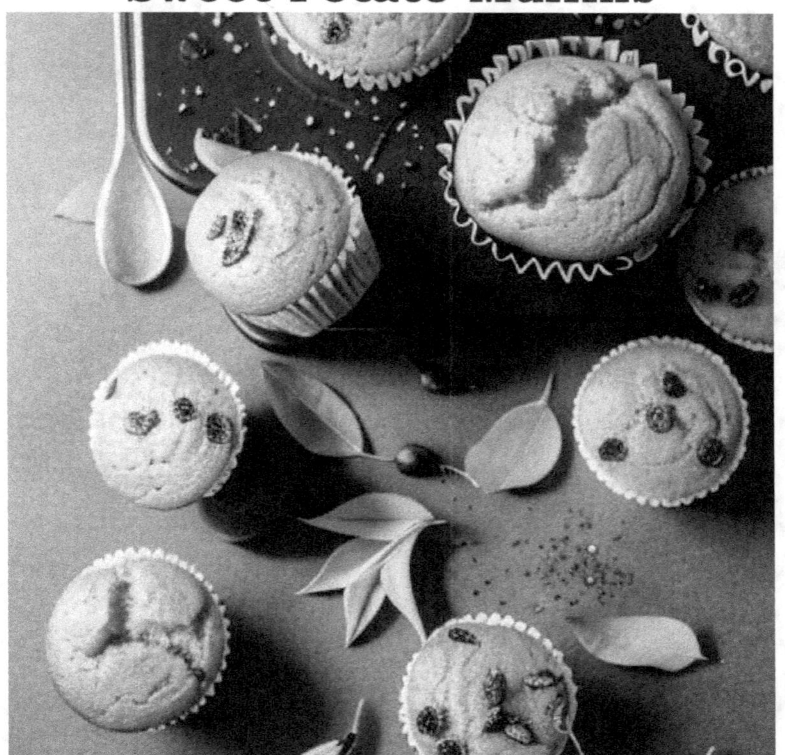

Ingredients:

- 2 cups mashed, cooked sweet potatoes
- 2 eggs.
- 1/4 cups of oil, 1 teaspoon vanilla,
- 1 cup of sugar, 2 teaspoons of baking soda, and 2 cups of all-purpose flour
- baking powder, 1 teaspoon

- 1/2 teaspoon of salt and 1 teaspoon of cinnamon powder
- 3/4 cups of walnuts, chopped (optional)

Instructions:

- First, preheat the oven to 350 degrees Fahrenheit.
- Spray cooking spray into muffin tins.
- Combine the mashed sweet potato, eggs, oil, and vanilla in a big bowl.
- Combine the flour, sugar, baking soda, baking powder, salt, and cinnamon in another bowl.
- Stirring gently to incorporate, gradually add the dry ingredients to the wet components.
- If using, fold in the chopped walnuts.
- Pour the batter into the muffin tins that have been prepared.
- Bake the cake for 25 to 30 minutes, or until the middle of the cake tester comes out clean.

Avocado Banana Smoothie

Ingredients:

- 1 ripe avocado
- a single ripe banana

- One cup of almond milk1 teaspoon each of ground cinnamon and honey

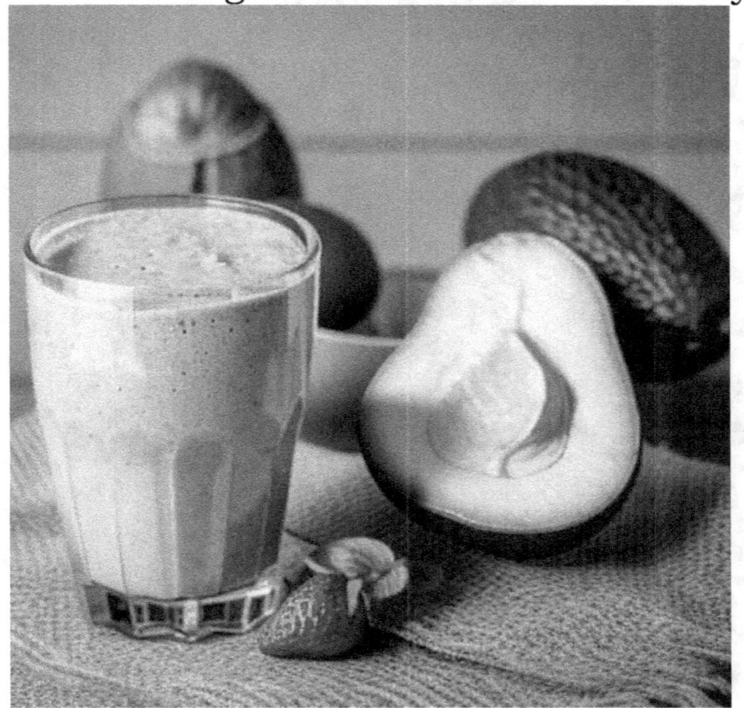

Instructions:

- The avocado should be peeled and pitted.
- Banana peeling
- Fill a blender with the avocado, banana, almond milk, honey, and cinnamon.
- Blend till fluid.
- Serve right away.

Fruit Pizza with Cream Cheese Frosting

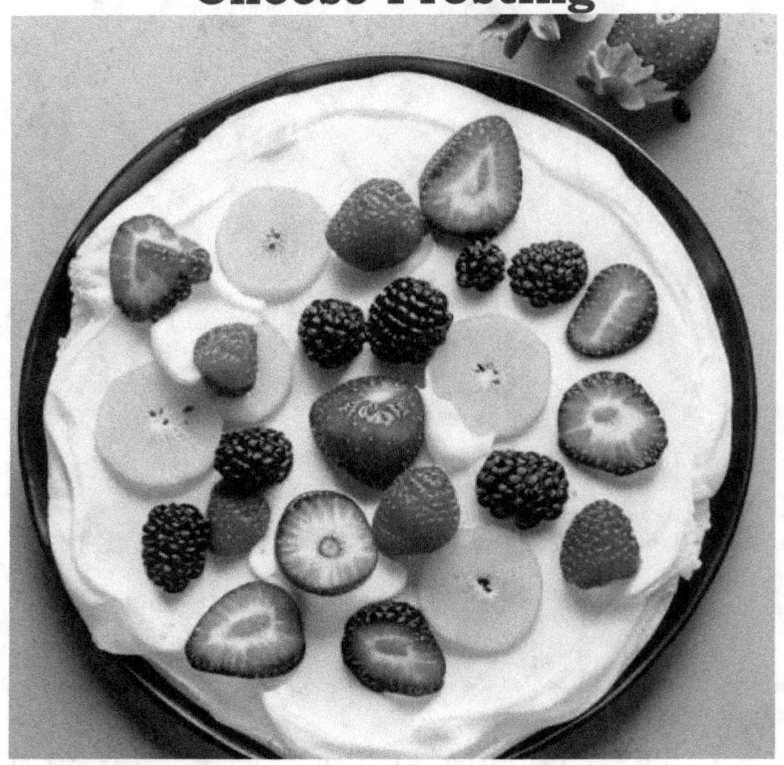

Ingredients

- one pre-baked 10-inch pizza crust, eight ounces of cream cheese
- one and a half cups of powdered sugar, and two teaspoons of orange juice.
- 2 teaspoons of melted butter
- One teaspoon vanilla

- 2 cups of mixed fresh fruit, such as blueberries, kiwis, and strawberries

Instructions:

- Set the oven's temperature to 350°F.
- Put the pizza crust on a baking sheet
- To create the frosting, combine the cream cheese, powdered sugar, melted butter, vanilla, and orange juice. Mix until smooth and frothy.
- Cover the crust with icing and top with a uniform layer of fruit.
- Bake the crust for 15 to 20 minutes, or until brown. Serve hot.

5-DAY MEAL PLAN

Day 1
Breakfast: Mediterranean Quinoa Salad
Lunch: Vegetable-or-Chicken Fajitas
Dinner: Baked Halibut with Tomato-Basil Salsa

Day 2
Breakfast: Southwest Chicken Chili
Lunch: Spinach-Stuffed Chicken Breasts
Dinner: Seared Tuna with Avocado Salsa

Day 3
Breakfast: Sweet Potatoes with Broccoli & Walnuts
Lunch: Grilled Asparagus & Orzo Salad
Dinner: Mediterranean Turkey Burgers

Day 4
Breakfast: Grilled Salmon with Lemon-Dill Sauce
Lunch: Steamed Vegetables with Garlic Sauce
Dinner: Quinoa-Stuffed Peppers

Day 5

Breakfast: Baked Salmon with Avocado Cream Sauce
Lunch: Zucchini Noodles with Mushroom Sauce
Dinner: Butternut Squash & Spinach Lasagna

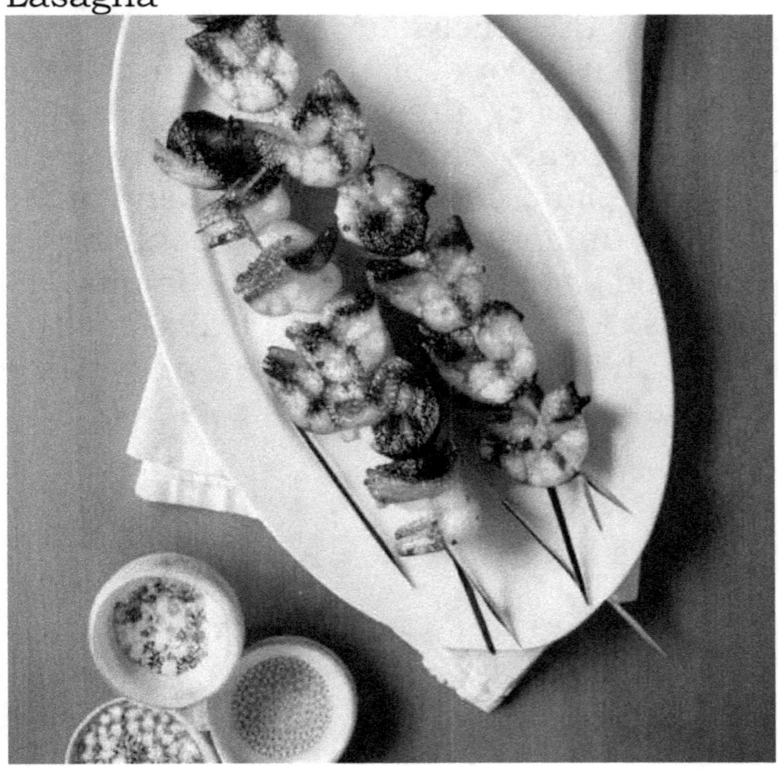

CONCLUSION

The Heart Disease Cookbook for Kids offers parents the opportunity to feed their kids scrumptious, wholesome, and heart-healthy food. It is crucial to protect and nourish the heart from an early age because it is one of the most important organs. Over time, preparing heart-healthy meals can aid in keeping your child's weight, cholesterol levels, and other factors under control. This cookbook is intended to motivate your family to increase the number of heart-healthy meals they eat each week. We appreciate your interest in reading this cookbook.

I'm grateful that you took the time to read my book. I hope you like it and it gave you something to think about. Thank You

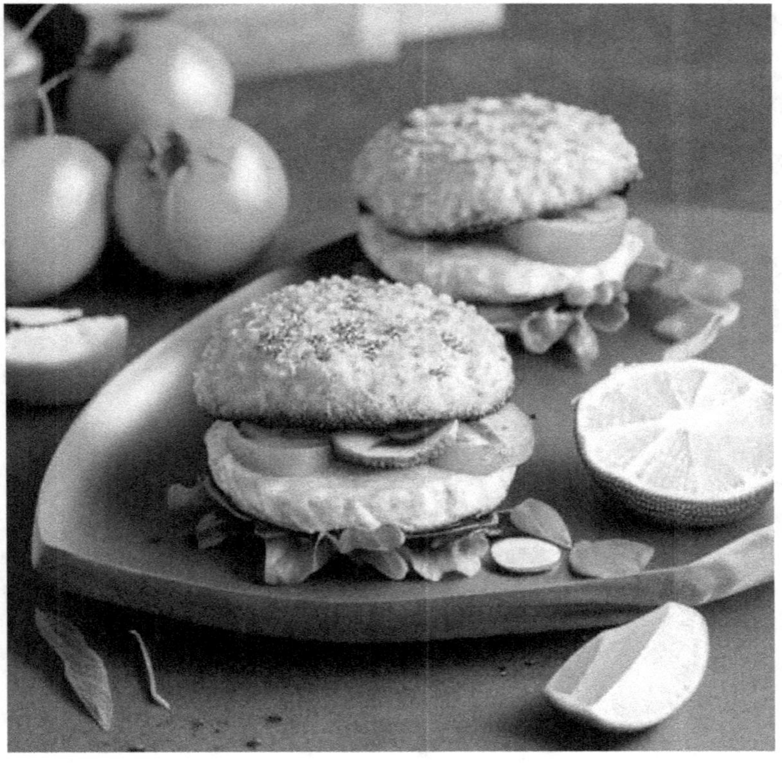

MEAL PLANNER

WEEK_________

MONDAY

BREAKFAST

LUNCH

DINNER

DESSERTS

SNACKS

TUESDAY

BREAKFAST

LUNCH

DINNER

____

____

DESSERTS

____

____

SNACKS

____

____

WENESDAY

BREAKFAST

____

____

LUNCH

____

____

DINNER

____

____

DESSERTS

____

____

SNACKS

THURSDAY

BREAKFAST

LUNCH

DINNER

DESSERTS

SNACKS

FRIDAY

BREAKFAST

LUNCH

DINNER

DESSERTS

SNACKS

SATURDAY

BREAKFAST

LUNCH

DINNER

DESSERTS

SNACKS

SUNDAY

BREAKFAST

LUNCH

DINNER

DESSERTS

SNACKS

NOTES

MONDAY

BREAKFAST
____
____

LUNCH
____
____

DINNER
____
____

DESSERTS
____
____

SNACKS
____
____

TUESDAY

BREAKFAST
____
____

LUNCH
____
____

DINNER

DESSERTS

SNACKS

WENESDAY

BREAKFAST

LUNCH

DINNER

DESSERTS

SNACKS

THURSDAY

BREAKFAST

LUNCH

DINNER

DESSERTS

SNACKS

FRIDAY

BREAKFAST

LUNCH

DINNER

DESSERTS

SNACKS

SATURDAY

BREAKFAST

LUNCH

DINNER

DESSERTS

SNACKS

____

____

SUNDAY

BREAKFAST

____

____

LUNCH

____

____

DINNER

____

____

DESSERTS

____

____

SNACKS

____

____

NOTES

____

____

____

____

WEEK__________

MONDAY

BREAKFAST

____

____

LUNCH

____

____

DINNER

____

____

DESSERTS

____

____

SNACKS

____

____

TUESDAY

BREAKFAST

____

____

LUNCH

____

____

DINNER

____

____

DESSERTS

____

____

SNACKS

____

____

WENESDAY

BREAKFAST

____

____

LUNCH

____

____

DINNER

____

____

DESSERTS

____

____

SNACKS

THURSDAY

BREAKFAST

LUNCH

DINNER

DESSERTS

SNACKS

FRIDAY

BREAKFAST

LUNCH

DINNER

DESSERTS

SNACKS

SATURDAY

BREAKFAST

LUNCH

DINNER

DESSERTS

SNACKS

____

____

SUNDAY

BREAKFAST

____

____

LUNCH

____

____

DINNER

____

____

DESSERTS

____

____

SNACKS

____

____

NOTES

____

____

____

____

MONDAY

BREAKFAST

____

____

LUNCH

____

____

DINNER

____

____

DESSERTS

____

____

SNACKS

____

____

TUESDAY

BREAKFAST

____

____

LUNCH

____

____

DINNER

____

____

DESSERTS

____

____

SNACKS

____

____

WENESDAY

BREAKFAST

____

____

LUNCH

____

____

DINNER

____

____

DESSERTS

____

____

SNACKS

THURSDAY

BREAKFAST

LUNCH

DINNER

DESSERTS

SNACKS

FRIDAY

BREAKFAST

LUNCH

DINNER

____

DESSERTS

____

SNACKS

____

SATURDAY

BREAKFAST

____

LUNCH

____

DINNER

____

DESSERTS

____

SNACKS

____

____

SUNDAY

BREAKFAST

____

LUNCH

____

DINNER

____

DESSERTS

____

SNACKS

____

NOTES

____

____

____

____

MONDAY

BREAKFAST

____

____

LUNCH

____

____

DINNER

____

____

DESSERTS

____

____

SNACKS

____

____

TUESDAY

BREAKFAST

____

____

LUNCH

____

____

DINNER

____

DESSERTS

____

____

SNACKS

____

____

WENESDAY

BREAKFAST

____

LUNCH

____

DINNER

____

DESSERTS

____

SNACKS

THURSDAY

BREAKFAST

LUNCH

DINNER

DESSERTS

SNACKS

FRIDAY

BREAKFAST

LUNCH

DINNER

DESSERTS

SNACKS

SATURDAY

BREAKFAST

LUNCH

DINNER

DESSERTS

SNACKS

____

____

SUNDAY

BREAKFAST

____

____

LUNCH

____

____

DINNER

____

____

DESSERTS

____

____

SNACKS

____

____

NOTES

____

____

____

____